I0439407

Lyme Disease Cookbook

*The definitive beginner's guide to healing
Lyme disease naturally*

Ben Plus Publishing

Table of Contents

Introduction

What Exactly Is Lyme Disease?

The Lyme Disease Diet

The Lyme Disease Diet

Gluten

Sugar

Nightshades

Dairy

Vitamin C

Meats, Protein and Energy

A Healthy Change

Breakfast Ideas

Lunch and Dinner Ideas

Snack Ideas

Introduction

It is the nature of a disease to produce unwanted effects such as discomfort to the sufferer. While pain is subjective, some diseases have been known to produce particularly painful or uncomfortable signs and symptoms. Lyme disease is one of them.

It might not be as popular as some dreaded diseases and conditions, but ask any Lyme disease sufferer and he or she will tell you all about the pain and discomfort that the disease brings. Lyme disease is a bacterial infection that causes a host of signs and symptoms, such as headaches, soreness of muscles, fever, and body malaise. A distinctive bull's eye-like rash appears in most cases, particularly the point of infection.

These signs and symptoms change and worsen as the infection settles in the body. Patients can experience meningitis, resulting in a severely painful stiff neck as well as light sensitivity. The heart and the brain can also become compromised, with sufferers having palpitations, memory loss, mood changes, and even sleep disturbances. Even in the earlier stages of the infection, Lyme disease causes all manners of pain through inflammation. These include pain in the joints, muscles, and tendons that tend to migrate to other places. There is also a condition known as radiculoneuritis, an inflammation of the nerves, which causes severe shooting pains that patients sometimes wake up from sleep.

More signs and symptoms follow during the late stages, but most of them could be prevented by seeking medical treatment, which is usually an aggressive round of antibiotics. However, even with early treatment of antibiotics, most of the inflammatory symptoms will manifest, bringing pain and discomfort that could interfere with the sufferer's daily activities, such as going to school, to work, or even with just going about one's daily routine around the house.

This is what those suffering from Lyme disease experience throughout the course of infection. The inflammatory attacks come in bursts, with no apparent cause, so patients could be fine in one moment and in pain the next. Most people will just suffer through them and keep a bottle of analgesics with them to take once the tendon, muscle, or joint pain starts attacking, but there are times when this is not very helpful, such as when attacks happen during sleep. Furthermore, it is not desirable for Lyme disease sufferers to consume analgesics while they are already burdening their system with strong antibiotics. The immune system is already shot due to the infection… must the patient add more chemicals to the mix?

What Exactly Is Lyme Disease?

For such a disease that causes severe pain and discomfort, it seems as if not much is known about it. What is Lyme disease, and how does it enter and affect the body?

Lyme disease is a bacterial infection that is mainly introduced to the body though a tick bite, though mosquitoes, lice, and fleas could potentially spread the infection as well, albeit to just a small degree. The bacteria in question are those from the *Borrelia* family, with specific types of the bacteria changing depending on the location. In North America, for example, most Lyme disease cases are caused by Borrelia burgdorferi, while in Europe, cases are mostly caused by Borrelia garinii and Borrelia afzelii. These bacteria are carried normally by hard ticks found in deer and mice in the wild, though there are rare cases of Lyme disease caught from particularly infested dogs and cats.

Once bitten, the bacteria will spread throughout the body, such as the joints, the heart, skin, and the peripheral and central nervous system. Unlike most bacteria, the *Borrelia* family are spirochetes—spiral-shaped organisms that can "hook" themselves onto the host cells. As such, these particular types of bacteria are harder to kill, requiring stronger mixes of antibiotics.

Because of this, the antibiotic treatment for Lyme disease could last for several weeks, and while this will kill the bacteria causing the infection, the body's immune system will keep on attacking the spirochetes, causing the inflammation, which in turn causes the pain and discomfort that sufferers experience. Also, since the spirochetes are present virtually everywhere, attacks are often described as "migrating" or "shooting".

Most people will rely on analgesics such as NSAIDs, or non-steroidal anti-inflammatory drugs to control the pain, but NSAIDs have their own side effects that could add to the discomfort of the Lyme disease patient. These include stomach upsets, heartburn, even gastritis.

This is one of the main reasons why naturalists or alternative medicine advocates and practitioners started rallying behind the Lyme disease diet—a natural and holistic way of boosting the immune system while suppressing the body's inflammatory response.

The Lyme Disease Diet

The disease is caused by an infection of bacterial spirochetes. The body responds to the infection and starts fighting off the bacteria. As a result, the surrounding cells become inflamed, causing pain.

To reduce the pain that makes the disease incredibly unbearable, an effective treatment should speed up the body's fight against the bacteria as well as minimizing the inflammation. Inflammation in itself is a natural body response, and is a crucial step in healing, but there are certain things that can exacerbate inflammation even more.

The Lyme disease diet addresses both points. This diet change aims to boost the immune system by choosing foods rich in vitamins and minerals, eliminating the biggest food culprits that cause or aggravate inflammation, as well as adding some herbs, leaves, and fruits that are known to soothe inflammation in the body.

Most Lyme disease diets advocate the following:

- Elimination of gluten-rich foods

- Elimination of sugar

- Elimination of foods from the nightshade family

- Elimination of dairy

- Elimination or limiting meats

- Increase of vitamin C-rich foods

Gluten

Gluten is a component—a protein—found in most grains and grain products. These include wheat, barley, rye, and its host of goods, such as breads, pasta, dough, and to some extent, alcoholic drinks like beer.

The concept of a Gluten-free diet is not in any way new; this kind of diet is also advised for persons suffering from wheat allergy and Celiac disease, a condition when the body cannot break down gluten, causing uncomfortable stomach upsets and other digestive problems. Due to the growing awareness of this disease, many restaurants and food companies have begun making gluten-free menus and products, so it is not difficult for a person suffering from Lyme disease to find gluten-free goods and restaurants.

Now, a person with Lyme disease might be able to break down gluten without problems, so why eliminate it from the diet? This is because in most cases of wheat allergy and Celiac disease, gluten-rich foods cause an allergic reaction—an inflammatory response. If the body already produces an inflammatory response due to the fight against the Borrelia bacteria, eating gluten might aggravate the condition, causing more painful attacks. Eliminating gluten from one's diet throughout the course of treatment is advised.

Most commercial products will have labels telling people which items are gluten-free, while restaurants will usually have a gluten-free menu. If possible, people can ask the waiters if there are any gluten-free choices available.

Sugar

Sugar is something that almost no one can hate. Sweet and mentally rewarding, almost every food item today contains sugar, be it breads, soups, meals, even drinks.

Of course, the most common examples of sugar-rich foods that should be avoided are cakes, pastries, ice cream, and soda, among others, but even certain fruits and berries contain high doses of fruit sugar known as fructose. These fruits, though they could give vitamins, minerals, and fiber, could also aggravate the disease.

Unlike gluten, which could aggravate the inflammation, sugar aggravates the disease by feeding the bacteria causing the disease. Bacteria feed on sugar, so a body with high blood sugar content would be like a feast for the spirochetes the body is trying to get rid of. Eliminating sugar from one's diet will starve the bacteria, weakening them, making them easier to defeat.

Aside from sugary treats and drinks, those who would like to follow the Lyme disease diet should also refrain from eating these fruits:

- Apples
- Apricots
- Bananas
- Blackberries
- Blueberries
- Cherries
- Grapes
- Kiwis
- Mangoes

- Oranges

- Pears

- Plums

- Raspberries

Nightshades

Nightshades are foods that are rich in alkaloids. As it turns out, alkaloids could impair nerve, muscle, and joint function—something Lyme disease sufferers do not need.

Foods that belong to the nightshade include:

- Cayenne
- Eggplants
- Paprika
- Pepinos
- Peppers, both hot and sweet
- Pimentos
- Potatoes (some doctors include sweet potatoes)
- Tabasco sauce
- Tamarios
- Tomatoes
- Tomatillos

Some doctors will allow moderate consumption of nightshade foods, as long as they are cooked thoroughly. The alkaloid content of nightshade foods lowers to around 40 to 50% from cooking. However, incredibly sensitive individuals, such as those who easily get heartburn or gastric upsets, should avoid eating these foods altogether.

Dairy

Aside from wheat and gluten, milk and dairy products are one other major source of food allergy. Allergies are basically the body's inflammatory response, so in the same way that gluten-rich foods are avoided, the same should be observed for this food group.

Now, some people might claim that they are not allergic or intolerant to milk and other lactose-rich food and drinks, but most dairy products contain the protein casein, which is derived from bovine milk. Casein causes and aggravates inflammation in most people.

Goat milk is said to contain lesser casein, but better alternatives are plant-derived milks, such as soy or almond milks.

Vitamin C

Vitamin C is well-known to bring nothing but good things to the body. Vitamin C boosts the immune system, so as the body becomes stronger against co-infections, it also becomes stronger to attack the harder to kill spirochetes.

Contrary to popular belief, foods that are rich in vitamin C are not limited to citrus fruits. In fact, most vitamin C-rich foods are vegetables.

Dark leafy greens such as broccoli, moringga, cabbages, collard greens, leeks, asparagus, spinach, kale, etc. are prime examples. These could be eaten raw or lightly steamed.

Aside from leafy greens, mushrooms also contain hefty amounts of vitamin C. Another bonus is that mushrooms are rich in protein, so those who are cutting meats could still get their protein from mushrooms.

Meats, Protein and Energy

Depending on the doctor, meats could be limited to a select few. Meats are rich in protein, but depending on the quality, could cause or aggravate inflammation.

Speaking of protein, people might wonder as to where they would get their energy, as most sources of sugar and carbohydrates are eliminated in the Lyme disease diet. Aside from carbohydrates, protein also gives the body the energy to burn, and there are a number of foods besides meats that are rich in protein. Mushroom was an example already given. Others include:

- Nuts

- Eggs

- Chia seeds

- Flax seeds

- Hemp seeds

- Beans and legumes

- Extra virgin coconut oil

- Extra virgin olive oil

- Raw and unfiltered apple cider vinegar

These foods are good examples of protein-rich foods. Aside from protein, oils from nuts, olives, and coconuts all contain anti-inflammatory properties, which mean they will help soothe the pain associated with Lyme disease.

Beans and legumes are also high in fiber, which will aid the body in eliminating toxins.

Chia, flax, and hemp seeds, aside from being rich in protein and vitamin C, are good alternatives for people who cook with Gluten-rich grains like wheat, rye and barley. There are many gluten-free recipes that call for these seeds in place of the gluten-rich grains to make breads, crackers, and all sorts of baked goods.

Apple cider vinegar is one food that is highly advocated by most naturalists. Aside from being rich in vitamin C, natural proteins, and in anti-inflammatory properties, apple cider vinegar also alkalizes food.

The concept of alkalizing acidic foods is also not new, but the simple explanation is that most diseases and conditions flourish in an acidic body. Bacteria like Borrelia are no exception—these organisms prefer acidic environments than alkaline ones. Lyme disease diet advocates claim that alkalizing the body will help weaken the bacteria.

A Healthy Change

Changing the diet in this way might appear drastic to some, but the pain associated with Lyme disease is no laughing matter, either. If sacrificing a few bad food choices could lead to a faster recovery and a healthier body, this kind of change is in no way difficult.

Lyme Disease Meal Ideas

Breakfast Ideas

Amazon Smoothie

Prep time: 5 minutes

INGREDIENTS

1 handful spinach

½ avocado

1 banana

1 large stalk celery

1 tsp cinnamon

1 cup water

INSTRUCTIONS

1. Slice avocado in half and remove the nut. Break the banana into small pieces and chop the celery into small pieces.
2. Combine all ingredients except for the spinach into a blender. Blend them until pureed, then add spinach and blend until pureed. Serve or chill and then serve.

Green Goodness Smoothie

Prep Time: 5 minutes

INGREDIENTS

2 cups spinach

2 whole kale leaves (1 cup chopped)

1 banana

1 green apple

1/2 cup green grapes

1 cup water (or fresh nut milk)

INSTRUCTIONS

1. Remove stems and ribs from kale. Core apple and dice. Peel banana.
2. Add water, banana and grapes to full sized blender. Process until solids are broken down.
3. Add greens and pulse on low for 30 seconds to break down. Then process on high for 1 minute, until smooth.
4. Pour into serving glasses and serve immediately.
5. Or chill in refrigerator for 20 minutes, blend for a few seconds to incorporate separated liquid, then pour into serving glasses and serve chilled.

Northern Typhoon

Prep time: 5 minutes

INGREDIENTS

1 handful Kale

1 banana

1 large cucumber

1 handful green beans

1 tsp cinnamon

1 cup water

INSTRUCTIONS

1. Break the banana into small pieces. De-stem the kale, skin and chop the cucumber and de-stem the green beans.
2. Combine all ingredients except for kale in a blender. Blend them until pureed, then add kale and blend until pureed. Serve or chill and then serve.

Pineapple Coconut Smoothie

Prep Time: 10 minutes*

INSTRUCTIONS

1 fresh coconut (or 1/2 cup flaked coconut)

1/2 cup pineapple chunks (fresh or frozen)

1 cup ice (crushed preferably)

Water

DIRECTIONS

1. *Soak flaked coconut in 1 1/2 cups water in refrigerator overnight, if using.

2. Add soaked coconut and soaking liquid to high-speed blender. Or remove flesh from fresh coconut and add to high-speed blender with 1 1/2 cups water. Process until well blended and fairly smooth, about 1 - 2 minutes.

3. Strain mixture through nut milk bag, cheesecloth or strainer back into blender.

4. Reserve pulp and set aside to dry and dehydrate, then use as coconut flour.

5. Cut pineapple flesh from peel, then chop. Add to blender with ice. Process until smooth, about 1 - 2 minutes.

6. Pour into serving glass and serve immediately.

Sweet Citrus Salad with Coconut Cream

Prep Time: 10 minutes

Servings: 1

INSTRUCTIONS

1 fresh coconut (or 1/2 cup flaked coconut)

1/4 - 1/3 cup dried pitted dates

1 blood orange

1 tangerine (or navel orange or clementine)

1/2 grapefruit (ruby red, pink or white)

1/2 lime

Water

INGREDIENTS

1. *Soak flaked coconut in 1 cup water overnight in refrigerator, if using. Soak dates in enough water to cover overnight in refrigerator. Drain.

2. Add soaked coconut and soaking liquid to high-speed blender. Or remove flesh from fresh coconut and add to high-speed blender with 3/4 cup water. Process until thick and fairly smooth, about 1 - 2 minutes.

3. Strain mixture through nut milk bag, cheesecloth or strainer back into blender or to food processor.

4. Reserve pulp and set aside to dry and dehydrate, then use as coconut flour.

5. Add soaked dates to processor and process until smooth. Set aside.

6. Peel all citrus and cut into segments. Add to serving dish. Top with sweet coconut cream.

7. Serve immediately. Or refrigerate 20 minutes and serve chilled.

Lunch and Dinner Ideas

Roasted Turkey Legs

Prep Time: 10 minutes*

Cook Time: 1 hour 20 minutes

Servings: 4

INGREDIENTS

2 large turkey legs

1/2 teaspoon garlic powder

1/2 teaspoon onion powder

1/2 teaspoon dried rosemary

1/2 teaspoon dried thyme

1/2 teaspoon Celtic sea salt

1 1/2 tablespoon coconut oil

Brine

4 cups water

1/4 cup Celtic sea salt

1/4 cup date butter

INSTRUCTIONS

1. *For *Brine*, add water, salt and date butter to wide, shallow container. Mix to combine. Add turkey legs and submerge completely in *Brine*. Marinate in refrigerator 12 - 24 hours.

2. Preheat oven to 350 degrees F. Place wire rack over sheet pan.

3. Remove turkey legs from brine. Rub salt, spices and oil over turkey legs, and under skin.

4. Place coated turkey legs on wire rack and bake about 35 - 40 minutes. Carefully turn turkey legs over and bake another 35 - 40 minutes, until skin is crisp and meat is cooked through.

5. Remove from oven and let rest about 2 minutes. Then serve hot.

Highland Beef Haggis

Prep Time: 10 minutes

Cook Time: 3 hours

Servings: 4

INGREDIENTS

8 oz (1/2 lb) ground beef (or bison, elk, etc.)

8 oz (1/2 lb) lamb shoulder

4 oz (1/4 lb) calves liver

2 onions (yellow or white)

1/2 head cauliflower (about 1 cup riced)

1 cup beef stock

2 garlic cloves

1/2 teaspoon ground nutmeg

1/4 teaspoon ground coriander

1/2 teaspoon Celtic sea salt

1/4 cup coconut oil

Water

INSTRUCTIONS

1. Preheat oven to 300 degrees F. Generously coat baking dish with coconut oil.

2. Add liver to small pan with enough water to cover over high heat. Bring to simmer and cook about 5 minutes. Drain and set aside to cool.

3. Roughly chop cauliflower. Peel and roughly chop onions and garlic. Add to food processor with lamb shoulder and par-cooked liver. Process until coarsely ground, about 2 minutes.

4. Add ground beef, stock, salt, and spices and pulse to combine. Transfer to prepared baking dish and cover tightly with aluminum foil.

5. Place covered dish in roasting pan. Add water to roasting pan 3/4 of the way up side of baking dish.

6. Bake for 3 hours. Remove from oven and carefully remove foil. Let rest about 10 minutes.

7. Remove baking dish from roasting pan. To plate, place serving dish over baking dish and carefully invert. Slice haggis into wedges and serve hot.

Bacon Wrapped Filet Mignon

Prep Time: 5 minutes

Cook Time: 20 minutes

Servings: 2

INGREDIENTS

2 (6 oz each) filet mignon steaks

2 thick slices nitrate-free bacon

Celtic sea salt, to taste

1 tablespoon coconut oil (optional)

Toothpicks

INSTRUCTIONS

1. Preheat oven to 350 degrees F. Heat medium oven-safe pan or skillet over medium heat.
2. Add bacon to hot pan. Cook and render out fat for about 5 minutes, until about halfway cooked. Remove bacon from pan and set aside, reserving bacon fat in pan. Add coconut oil to pan, if desired.
3. Wrap par-cooked bacon around steaks and secure with toothpick. Sprinkle steaks with salt to taste.
4. Add wrapped seasoned steaks to hot oiled pan and sear 2 minutes per side. Carefully flip half way through cooking.
5. Remove pan from stove and place in preheated oven. Cook about 8 - 10 minutes, until bacon is cooked through and steak is medium-rare.
6. Remove steaks from oven and transfer to cutting board. Set aside and let rest at least 2 minutes.

7. Transfer to serving dish and serve hot.

Herb Roasted Pork Tenderloin

Prep Time: 10 minutes*

Cook Time: 15 minutes

Servings: 4

INGREDIENTS

1 pork tenderloin

1 teaspoon dried rosemary

1 teaspoon dried thyme

1 teaspoon dried oregano

1 teaspoon dried basil

1 teaspoon dried marjoram (optional)

1 teaspoon Celtic sea salt

Apricot Sauce

1 cup dried apricots

2/3 cup water

1 teaspoon apple cider vinegar (or dry white wine)

INSTRUCTIONS

1. Preheat oven to 425 degrees F. Heat small pan over medium heat.
2. Rub tenderloin with salt and spices, then press into meat so it adheres. Place on sheet pan, or wire rack over sheet pan.
3. Roast for 10 - 15 minutes, until just cooked through and no pink remains. Remove pork from oven and let rest 10 minutes.

4. For *Apricot Sauce*, add dried apricots, water and vinegar to food processor or high-speed blender. Process until smooth, about 1 - 2 minutes.

5. Add *Apricot Sauce* to hot pan and reduce until slightly thickened. Stir well and do not let burn. Remove from heat.

6. Slice pork and transfer to serving dish. Top pork with *Apricot Sauce* and serve warm.

Classic Churrasco with Chimichurri

Prep Time: 10 minutes*

Cook Time: 5 minutes

Servings: 4

INGREDIENTS

24 oz (1 1/2 lb) beef tenderloin

Chimichurri

1 cup coconut oil

1/3 cup apple cider vinegar (or coconut aminos)

1/3 cup water

1 large bunch cilantro

1 large bunch parsley

1/2 cup fresh mint leaves

6 garlic cloves

1 teaspoon Celtic sea salt

INSTRUCTIONS

1. For *Chimichurri*, peel garlic and add to food processor or high-speed blender. Remove cilantro, parsley and mint leaves from stems. Add to processor and process to finely chop, about 1 minute. Add oil, water, salt and spices. Process until thick sauce forms, about 1 - 2 minutes.

2. Cut tenderloin lengthwise into 4 even slices, then flatten with tenderizing or kitchen mallet to 1/2 inch thickness. Place meat in between two parchment sheets to flatten, if preferred.

3. *Pour 1/4 of the *Chimichurri* into a baking dish just large enough to fit tenderloin. Place beef over *Chimichurri*, then top with second 1/4 of *Chimichurri*. Set aside to marinate about 1 hour. Transfer remaining *Chimichurri* to serving dish.
4. Heat grill or grated skillet over high heat.

Moist Roasted Turkey

Prep Time: 10 minutes*

Cook Time: 4 - 6 hours

Servings: 12

INGREDIENTS

20 lb (approx.) whole turkey

2 teaspoons Celtic sea salt

2 tablespoons coconut oil

Brine

1 - 2 gallons water

1 cup Celtic sea salt

1 cup date butter

INSTRUCTIONS

1. *For *Brine*, add 1/2 gallon of water, salt and date butter to large baking dish or roasting pan. Mix to combine. Remove any entrails from turkey and add to *Brine*, plus and enough water to submerge completely. Marinate in refrigerator 12 - 24 hours.

2. Preheat oven to 350 degrees F. Place roasting rack in clean roasting pan.

3. Drain turkey and rub salt and oil over and under skin, where possible.

4. Place seasoned turkey on roasting rack and bake about 15 - 18 minutes per lb, about 5 hours for 20 lb bird. Or until internal

temperature reaches 165 degrees F. Baste with rendered fat and juices throughout cooking for even browning.

5. Remove turkey from oven and let rest 20 - 30 minutes.
6. Carve and serve warm.

Quick Raw Avocado Slaw

Prep Time: 10 minutes*

Cook Time: 20 minutes

Servings: 4

INGREDIENTS

1/2 head cabbage (2 cups shredded)

1 avocado

1 carrot

Zest of 1 lemon

Juice of 1 lemon

1 tablespoon raw honey

2 tablespoons apple cider vinegar

1 teaspoon sea salt

INSTRUCTIONS

1. Cut avocado in half and remove pit. Scoop flesh into large mixing bowl and mash with fork.
2. Remove any tough outer leaves and core from cabbage. Shred cabbage and carrot. Add to bowl with vinegar, honey and salt. Zest *then* juice lemon, and add.
3. Toss to combine.
4. Serve immediately. Or and place in refrigerator for 20 minutes and serve chilled.

Snack Ideas

Smoked Salmon and Avocado Snack

Prep Time: 5* minutes

Servings: 2

INGREDIENTS

4 oz (1 or 1/2 package) cold-smoked salmon

1 avocado

1 stalk fresh dill

Pinch sea salt

1/2 lemon (optional)

INSTRUCTIONS

1. Slice avocado in half and remove pit. Cut into thick slices in peel then scoop out with large spoon.
2. Slice smoked salmon into long 1 inch strips. Wrap 1 salmon strips around each avocado slice. Arrange wrapped avocado on serving dish.
3. Mince fresh dill. Sprinkle dill and salt over avocado wraps and serve immediately.
4. Or squeeze juice of 1/2 lemon over avocado wraps, sprinkle on dill and salt, and refrigerate 20 minutes. Then serve chilled.

Olive Tapenade

Prep Time: 15 minutes

Servings: 2

INGREDIENTS

1 1/2 cups any combination pitted olives (Kalamata, Spanish, black, pimento, etc.)

2 tablespoons capers

2 anchovy fillets

1 garlic clove

2 fresh basil leaves

1/2 lemon

2 tablespoons coconut oil

INSTRUCTIONS

1. Peel garlic and add to food processor or high-speed blender. Process until finely ground.
2. Rinse and drain olives, capers and anchovy fillets. Add to processor with basil, oil and squeeze of 1/2 lemon. Process until finely chopped or coarsely ground, about 1 - 2 minutes.
3. Transfer to serving dish and serve immediately.

Spicy Tuna Tartare

Prep Time: 15* minutes

Servings: 4

INGREDIENTS

1 lb tuna steak (sushi grade)

1 small cucumber

1 ripe avocado

1 lime

1 garlic clove

2 tablespoons raw virgin coconut oil

Small bunch fresh cilantro

1 teaspoon sea salt

INSTRUCTIONS

1. Peel, seed and dice cucumber and avocado. Finely chop cilantro. Add to medium mixing bowl.
2. Remove seeds, stem and veins from hot pepper. Peel garlic and add to food processor or bullet blender. Process until smooth paste forms. Add to bowl.
3. Dice tuna, discarding any tough white gristle. Add to bowl.
4. Squeeze on lime juice and add salt.
5. Gently toss with soft spatula or large spoon.
6. Serve immediately. Or refrigerate 20 minutes and serve chilled.

Baked Candied Yams

Prep Time: 10 minutes

Cook Time: 1 hour 30 minutes

Servings: 12

INGREDIENTS

4 large sweet potatoes (yams)

1/2 cup dried pitted dates

1/4 cup dried apricots

2 tablespoons coconut butter

1 tablespoon ground cinnamon

1/2 teaspoon ground ginger

Pinch Celtic sea salt

Topping

1/4 cup date butter

INSTRUCTIONS

1. Preheat oven to 350 degrees F.
2. Gently rinse sweet potatoes and place on sheet pan.
3. Bake about 1 hour, until tender.
4. Add dates, apricots and enough water to cover in small pot. Heat over medium heat. Let simmer until water evaporates. Remove from heat.
5. Remove yams from oven and let cool about 10 minutes.

6. For *Topping*, add date butter to small pan. Heat over medium heat and cook for about 4 - 5 minutes. Stir frequently and do not burn. Remove from heat and set aside.

7. Add softened dates and apricots to large mixing bowl. Mash with potato masher, hand mixer or whisk.

8. Cut yams open lengthwise and scoop flesh into mixing bowl. Add butter, salt and spices. Mash with potato masher, hand mixer or whisk until well combined.

9. Transfer yam mixture to serving dish and top with *Topping*. Serve warm.

Lean Mean Collard Greens

Prep Time: 15 minutes

Cook Time: 2 1/2 hours

Servings: 8

INGREDIENTS

2 heads (or 2 large bags) fresh collard greens

6 slices nitrate-free bacon (or 1 small ham hock)

8 cups chicken stock

Water

INSTRUCTIONS

1. Preheat oven to 350 degrees F. Heat large pot over medium-high heat.
2. Rinse collards well and roughly chop. Place in large colander or in clean sink to drain.
3. Add bacon or ham hock to hot pot and render down for about 5 minutes.
4. Add greens to pot in batches. If all greens to not fit, reserve. Add chicken stock.
5. Bring pot to a simmer then reduce to low heat. Add any remaining greens, plus enough water just to cover, if necessary. Stir gently.
6. Simmer until collards are tender, about 2 - 2 1/2 hours.
7. Drain greens well. Transfer to serving dish and serve warm.

5. Place beef on grill or skillet on the diagonal and cook for about 1 minute, then rotate meat to create crosshatch grill marks and cook

for another minute. Then flip and repeat. Cook for about 4 minutes total for medium rare.

6. Remove from grill, slice against the grain and transfer to serving dish. Serve immediately with *Chimichurri*.

Turkey Jerky Bacon

Prep Time: 10 minutes*

Dehydrating Time: 4 - 8 hours

Servings: 4

INGREDIENTS

4 oz organic turkey (dark meat)

2 tablespoons coconut aminos (or liquid aminos)

2 tablespoons tamari (or liquid aminos or coconut aminos)

1 tablespoon lemon juice (or raw apple cider vinegar)

1 tablespoons Celtic sea salt

1/2 teaspoon garlic powder

1/2 teaspoon onion powder

INSTRUCTIONS

1. Prepare two sheet parchment. Lay one on cutting board.
2. Cut turkey into 1/4 inch strips and lay in single layer on parchment. Pound with tenderizing side of kitchen mallet. Cover turkey with second parchment sheet, then pound with flat side of tenderizing mallet to 1/8 inch thickness.
3. *Place turkey strips in medium mixing bowl or shallow dish. Add coconut aminos, tamari, lemon juice, salt and spices. Mix well to coat. Cover and place in refrigerator for 8 hours, or overnight.
4. Remove turkey from refrigerator and lay in single layer on dehydrator trays. Place trays in dehydrator and set to 120 degrees F for 4 - 8 hours.

5. After 4 hours dehydrating time, remove trays from dehydrator and test turkey by bending. If it cracks, remove and serve immediately. Or store in airtight container.

6. If still flexible, place back in dehydrator and continue dehydrating up to 4 hours, or until desired texture is achieved.

www.ingramcontent.com/pod-product-compliance
Lightning Source LLC
Chambersburg PA
CBHW070448290526
45791CB00005B/2096